Aloe Vera:

The Green Golden Magic

The Wonder that Aloe Vera is in Ayurveda

Anand Gupta

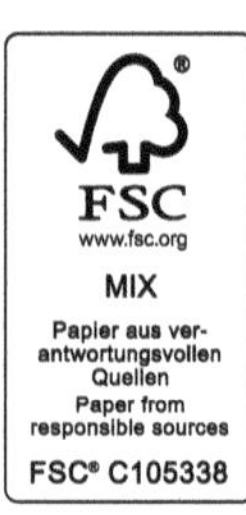

Bibliografische Information der Deutschen Nationalbibliothek:

Die Deutsche Nationalbibliothek verzeichnet diese Publikation in der Deutschen Nationalbibliografie; detaillierte bibliografische Daten sind im Internet über http://dnb.dnb.de abrufbar.

Herstellung und Verlag: BoD – Books on Demand, Norderstedt

ISBN: 978-3-7526-5800-2

Introduction

By using this book, you accept this disclaimer in full.

No advice

The book contains information. The information is not advice and should not be treated as such.

No representations or warranties

To the maximum extent permitted by applicable law and subject to section below, we exclude all representations, warranties, undertakings and guarantees relating to the book.

Without prejudice to the generality of the foregoing paragraph, we do not represent, warrant, undertake or guarantee:

- that the information in the book is correct, accurate, complete or non-misleading.

- that the use of the guidance in the book will lead to any particular outcome or result.

Limitations and exclusions of liability

6

The limitations and exclusions of liability set out in this section and elsewhere in this disclaimer: are subject to section 6 below; and govern all liabilities arising under the disclaimer or in relation to the book, including liabilities arising in contract, in tort (including negligence) and for breach of statutory duty.

We will not be liable to you in respect of any losses arising out of any event or events beyond our reasonable control.

We will not be liable to you in respect of any business losses, including without limitation loss of or damage to profits, income, revenue, use, production, anticipated savings, business, contracts, commercial opportunities or goodwill.

We will not be liable to you in respect of any loss or corruption of any data, database or software.

We will not be liable to you in respect of any special, indirect or consequential loss or damage.

Exceptions

Nothing in this disclaimer shall: limit or exclude our liability for death or personal injury resulting from negligence; limit or exclude our liability for fraud or fraudulent misrepresentation; limit any of our liabilities in any way that is not permitted under applicable law; or exclude any of our liabilities that may not be excluded under applicable law.

Severability

If a section of this disclaimer is determined by any court or other competent authority to be unlawful and/or unenforceable, the other sections of this disclaimer continue in effect.

If any unlawful and/or unenforceable section would be lawful or enforceable if part of it were deleted, that part will be deemed to be deleted, and the rest of the section will continue in effect.

Law and jurisdiction

This disclaimer will be governed by and construed in accordance with Swiss law, and any disputes relating to this disclaimer will be subject to the exclusive jurisdiction of the courts of Switzerland.

Inhaltsverzeichnis

Conclusion: 45

Introduction

"It was misty… wind was blowing the fog and clouds here and there. The green carpet beneath her feet was crunching and tickling her bare soles with its fronds. The dew drops making her shiver with the coldness, trees with tops so high, she couldn't see them; where was she?

Her hair was whipping across her face in the gusts of wind. She could not remember where she started from, how she got here in this mystical land of wonderment! As she walked on the sloping ground, she could see fairies swirling in the space ahead of her, in a green glow of the magical nature. What a sight!

Suddenly, they saw her! The three fairies flew straight at her with delight in their welcoming eyes. She was not scared, just a little-taken aback – was this a dream? And then she saw where the green glow was coming from. The fairy handed it to her and she just looked and looked, mesmerized. She knew it was a magically effective plant type since she had seen her mother using it for so many purposes, but this? She could now see the fairies were immortal because of the mysterious green, glowing plant leaves. What was it?

It was a frond from the Aloe Vera plant. It had been here; all this time."

We have all some time or the other in life, experienced the magic of nature. It helps us realize that whatever we are, however healthy, happy and content, is all because of the abundant gifts of nature itself. We freely utilize them, mostly taking it for granted and not even acknowledging the wonderful gifts we are endowed with. One such gift amongst the many is Aloe Vera – the plant with a multitude of qualities which makes life bit easier for us. Many problems of the body can be cured using Aloe Vera – the most commonly occurring, and most useful plant of the genus.

Let us read on in this e-book dedicated to Aloe Vera and understand the various uses or practical applications of the plant in Ayurveda, the ancient Indian medical science which uses natural ingredients after a lot of research for curing the disease organically and safely. This book intends to bring about an awareness regarding the plant and its everyday uses for medicinal benefits. We hope this book becomes a lucid and interesting read as well as guide you in terms of usage of the plant and its products. Enjoy your read!

Chapter 1:
About Aloe Vera – the plant of immortality

Who wants to die? We all want to live a long, prosperous and healthy life full of comfort and happiness. We are all looking for ways to be better in all aspects, to be safe and secure. We are aware of death and its consequences but we are constantly negating it, we like to think expansive. But in this life, there may be quite a few ups and downs, fitness and illness, Health and sickness. For every query, Ayurveda has a simple solution.

Aloe Vera is a truly mesmerizing plant. There are many ancient recordings where this plant has been put to use in dire situations and it turned the tide. Since Egyptian civilization (the oldest most sophisticated civilization) Aloe Vera has been used to various requirements. They also buried Aloe Vera with a Pharaoh in his pyramid so that it would continue to benefit him even in afterlife. Here are some interesting facts regarding Aloe Vera:

- In about 240 species in the Aloe family, only 4 are useful for medicinal properties. There are poisonous varieties too!
- This plant belongs to the lily family, but in appearance resembles the cactus!
- The leaves are used for all the benefits, and they are succulent, with tiny spikes on the edges. They are broad at the base and pointed at the tips. The leaves are a storehouse of clear gel which has all the medicinal properties. It is found that the gel contains 96% water and as many as 75 other components like minerals, vitamins, enzymes and 7 out of the 8 essential amino acids needed by the body.
- This plant is native to Spain and Africa. But these days this plant grows well in

Asia, Europe, and America but only the hot, dry regions.

- The plant does not have a prominent stem, one can rather say it is stem-less and it propagates through offset shoots.
- This plant is well adapted to aridness and lack of water. Thus, it becomes an ideal plant to grow in deserts, rocky places and even in themes gardens.
- The plant stores water in its leaves and so they are thick and fleshy.
- Aloe Vera may die due to over-watering or lack of drainage from the soil they have been put in.

In Ayurveda, this plant has a huge importance. Aloe Vera is a potent ayurvedic drug and used for many internal and external applications. It is considered a master component in all treatments concerning healing, rejuvenation and the like.

Kerala is often considered the home of Ayurveda and one can notice how common Aloe vera plant is in any home garden. For many years now, Aloe Vera has become a household herb and effective alternative medicine for the masses and classes alike.

Chapter 2: Uses of Aloe Vera in Ayurveda

Aloe vera finds many applications in ayurvedic practices. To understand the use better, let's look at the philosophy of Ayurveda and derivate the ways in which it works:

- Basic principle of Ayurveda is to find a balance between physical, spiritual, mental and even social wellbeing.
- It considers everything in the universe to be made up of identical five elements – water, air, earth, fire, and spirit. We are always connected to the universe and balanced connection brings good health.
- Any disorder or disease is caused by disruption in balance, which makes our body easily susceptible to infection or falling ill. Balance is disturbed by the

choices we make, voluntarily or involuntarily.

- Rather than curing the disease and related discomfort, Ayurveda aims at keeping the disease at bay, or prevention of illness itself. It propagates balanced behavior and habits so that there is no loss of harmony in the first place. There is more emphasis on preventive medicine than curative medicine. Preventive medicine finds out the person's "prakruti" and suggests a way of life so that the balance is maintained. Curative medicine focuses on a disease when it has already started to affect the person. Curative medicine is a highly method based and comprehensive branch, using lots of Ayurveda applications.

- There are many branches of ayurvedic science, dealing with various forms of healing like oral medicines, surgery, child medicine, chemistry and pharmacology, sexology, psychology, and psychiatry, etc.

Aloe vera finds use in various medicines as base ingredient as well as many direct applications are also equivalent to medicines, so Aloe Vera can be rightly considered the wondrous magical herb!

Most of us have seen the Aloe Vera plant as a component of our garden. It is called "ghritkumari" in Sanskrit, the language of Ayurveda. We have also noticed the thick, fleshy leaves being cut up and the gel and sap inside used for variety of uses. Let us take a look on how Aloe Vera is being used for the past hundreds of years, in Ayurveda and otherwise.

Aloe vera is useful as:

1. **For the gastro-intestinal tract**

- Bhedhani – relieves constipation
- Gulmhara – abdominal tumor relief
- Vatahara – gas and constipation relieving, deflates bloating
- Pleehahara – helpful in spleen related issues
- Vishahara – anti-poison and antitoxin

2. **For the female reproductive system**

- Granthihara – remedies fibroids and lymphadenitis in uterus
- Raktapittahara – helps control heavy bleeding (especially during periods)

3. **For skin problems –**

- Tvak roga – cures psoriasis
- Agnidagdha – helps heal burn wounds

- Visphotahara – provides relief from boils and blisters.
- Rasayana – anti ageing properties make it good for the skin health.

4. For general health issues

- Kapha jwarhara – fever treatment
- Balya – an enhancer for immunity
- Shwasahara – good for the respiratory system especially for asthma patients
- Yakrut vruddhihara – hepatitis relief/hepatomegaly cure
- Pittaja kasahara – cough and cold relief

5. For the eyes –

- Chakshushya – used in eye disorders and makes eyesight better

6. For the reproductive organs –

- Vrushya – improves vigor and considered aphrodisiac

7. **For joints –**

   - Vatahara – ati inflammatory properties

Aloe Vera benefits for the skin:

We are all conscious of the external appearance, and a good, healthy skin is one of the most coveted dreams of most of us. We all want radiant and healthy skin from within and for this Aloe Vera is quite an effective agent. These days many cosmetics use Aloe Vera in some form for the extraordinary advantages it provides.

- Great moisturizer – Aloe Vera is the life of any moisturizer because of the slippery gel which traps moisture and keeps it intact. This gel does not let the epithelium (uppermost layer of the skin) dry out or lose moisture and keeps it hydrated.

- Makes the skin look young and fresh - the sap, when applied on the skin, makes it smooth, fresh and well moisturized. The fact that the moisture is not lost makes the skin radiant and keeps it young for longer.

- Fights acne and keeps the face clear – the various good chemicals in Aloe Vera make it an ideal substance to fight acne. When applied in a face pack, the effect is miraculous and it even clears off the acne scars.

- Soothing for the skin – a face pack of Aloe Vera is bound to soothe sunburn and heal the ski rapidly. It is generally quite mild and reduces skin irritation. Thus, it is also helpful for allergies.

- When skin gets burnt in some accident and there is pain and irritation, Aloe Vera is the most potent ayurvedic medicine which will immediately bring relief, accelerate the skin regeneration pace and cure the burn faster. In accidents and kitchen related burns, Aloe Vera brings relief to the patient while healing the wound. The unique air locking properties of the gel also makes sure the wound does not form crust or dry out. The gel keeps the moisture in and air out. This makes way for a mark free healing of burn wound.

- Good skin is a sign of healthy body. Aloe vera is taken internally, as in, ingested for better gastro-intestinal function and liver health and this in total reflects on the skin. Thus, we can say Aloe Vera makes skin look more radiant and healthy.

- Scalp skin is also benefited by Aloe Vera, as it hydrates the scalp, removing dandruff, making hair shine and improving the general health of the scalp. It can also be applied on the hair as a conditioner to make them shiny and smooth.

Aloe Vera benefits for the digestive system:

Aloe vera is a wonder plant – the miracle maker which has many health advantages. No wonder, it is also excellent for the stomach and digestive health. Here is how:

- Aloe Vera is exceptionally good for the gastro-intestinal tract. When ingested, it relives constipation as it is a mild laxative and helps easy movement of food through the gut. It also soothes the stomach and intestine walls and removes any straining of the muscles of the tract.

- When one is suffering from ulcers and heartburn (the regurgitation of stomach acids into the esophagus or the food pipe, burning and hurting all the delicate tissues in the process and causing severe burning sensation), it can be very beneficial to drink Aloe juice. The compound has anti-inflammatory properties and is thus helpful.

- For liver enlargement, generally known to medical science as hepatomegaly, Aloe is quite helpful. It soothes the disorder and helps restore the liver to original size.

- Consuming Aloe is good for stomach lesions too. It also removes ulcerative colitis of the stomach.

Aloe vera benefits for immune system:

- The polysaccharides in Aloe Vera make it a very potent immunity booster. This property also makes it a great anti-tumor agent.
- The combination of the two creates a unique property of immunity provision as well as curing cancer as it is anti-cancer in nature.
- The abundance of minerals in Aloe Vera gel and juice also makes it good for immunity.

Aloe vera benefits for female and male reproductive organs:

- Aloe vera is an agent for better reproductive health for both men and women. It is found to be good for ovulation, cleansing the uterus during menstruation and thus used for amenorrhea.

- For men, this is an aphrodisiac and improves the sperm count by stimulating sperm production. It also increases the vigor in men.

Aloe vera benefits for diabetes:

Diabetes affects nearly 30% of the world population today, thanks to our sedentary, inactive lifestyle and poor dietary habits. The world is becoming a poor-digestion population and all we can think of is expensive medication like insulin shots and what not. Why not try ayurvedic medication like Aloe Vera to control and counter diabetes? Aloe vera has been found to be great for diabetes because:

- It improves the circulation and thus diabetic numbness is reduced significantly.

- It is shown to affect the blood sugar levels. People drinking Aloe Vera juice on a daily basis ted to have lesser fasting blood sugar levels.

Aloe vera benefits for arthritis:

Arthritis is a complicated disorder of the joints where there is inflammation in the joints and excruciating pain makes everyday work a challenge. The pain and discomfort even inhibit the patient to move about and finish one's routine activities. Modern day medicines mostly focus on the pain aspect of arthritis and pain killers are administered. Ayurveda focuses on eliminating the swelling itself and Aloe Vera helps in the following ways.

- Arthritis is actually inflammation of joints, and the anti-inflammatory capacities of Aloe make it ideal for relief from arthritis pain.

- Topical application is quite effective if you combine it with a suitable diet. Also, many a times ingestion is also recommended, if you are not sensitive to the laxative quality of Aloe Vera.

- If taken internally, make sure you eat a balanced diet with less fiber for maintaining stomach equilibrium.

Aloe vera benefits for cholesterol:

High cholesterol is like a silent killer. It will just keep clogging the arteries and make blood flow a challenge and one might not even know till it starts affecting the heart. One may have high cholesterol due to bad diet, lack of exercise or it may be hereditary. Whatever may be the reason, Aloe Vera is such a potent herb which lies at the hands of

Ayurveda and it can positively affect the patient.

- Aloe vera, when ingested, has shown to lower the triglycerides in blood and improve the quality of blood.
- Cholesterol is also reduced, and one can think about stopping the statin drugs completely if the Aloe Vera suits them.
- Combined with blueberry, this herb is bound to treat cholesterol issue effectively, so much so that one ca taper off the synthetic and harmful statin drugs for the same use.

So we see Aloe vera has a lot to offer! Being applicable in so many areas of health and wellness is wonderment in itself. That is why we call Aloe Vera a "miracle" plant.

It has been found that Aloe Vera is completely safe to ingest or apply. But there are certain hygiene factors one must consider before using Aloe Vera as an alternative medicine. We shall see them in the coming chapters.

Chapter 3:
Recipes and medicines of Aloe Vera, as per Ayurveda

Ayurveda being an ancient medical science developed in India talks much about Aloe Vera as it has been experimented widely and much good effect has been seen over the centuries. Some useful medicines and recipes including Aloe Vera are given below. But, one must definitely take a moment to check with one's doctor to make sure it is fine to use them with one's existing medication. Apart from taking juice and gel of Aloe Vera internally and applying topically, one can find these medicines and applications of Aloe vera in Ayurveda:

- Kumarayasav – used in various stomach ailments and colds as well. Piles is said to be cured by this medicine.

- Raja Pravartini Vati – used in treating amenorrhea or lack of periods in women and also scant periods.

- Mukta Panchamrit Ras – used in the treatment of fevers and cold.

- Karutha Gulika – used in treatment of headaches.

- Aloe vera in preparing Bhasma – a mixture of copper dust and Aloe Vera is used for variety of ailments like arthritis and sexual disorders.

- Face pack for anti-ageing – a mixture of Aloe Vera, olive oil and oatmeal makes your skin youthful and fresh.

- For acne and scars – mix some Aloe Vera in lemon juice and apply on the pimple. Leave it overnight and see the magical effect the other day.

- For hair growth and bald patch control – mix Aloe Vera gel in castor oil and apply topically on the affected areas. Leave it overnight and wash hair the next day.

- For better gastric health – mix some fresh or processed Aloe Vera gel with honey and water and consume the juice for good results. Only, the ones with a sensitive system should not use this juice as it is laxative in nature.

- Aloe vera juice can effectively cure GERD, blood sugar regulation and better the liver.

- Oral health concoction – for better teeth and gums, use Aloe Vera like toothpaste. Also, if one has dry mouth condition, Aloe juice as well as topical application is a great way to restore mouth hydration.

- Eye tonic – Aloe Vera is also good for the eyes, thanks to the various vitamins and minerals in the gel. It also soothes out any irritation that may cause damage to the eye, like a foreign substance or parti-cle or a chemical droplet. It is like a boon for tired eyes. One can directly apply some gel on the eyes and lie down for a few minutes.

Chapter 4:
Things to keep in mind

Aloe Vera is understandably a very versatile plant and is used in a wide variety of health issues. But since there is no thumb rule in Ayurveda, that is, nothing is uniform or similar for everyone, and treatments, effects, and dosages for every person are different, Aloe can be slightly different in effect for each one. It would be good if we keep the following points in mind before we use it on ourselves or someone else.

- Never administer a pregnant woman or a lactating new mother with ingestible Aloe Vera. Its properties which are otherwise quite helpful and effective might be a little too much for a delicate stage body like that of pregnancy.

- Aloe Vera may cause abdominal cramping or even diarrhea in some people. Since it is a laxative, it may not settle well for some people.

- First, test for reactivity in your body and then begin to use on a regular basis. If it does not suit you, you might get a slight rash in the worst case, or itchiness, redness or other similar mild symptoms.

- The latex of Aloe is quite an undesirable substance. When ingested in large amounts it can also become lethal so one must beware of it. It can cause hematuria too. One can avoid using the latex – it comes right under the plant's skin and can be seen yellowish in color.

- Aloe latex is also found to cause cancer!

- If using commercial Aloe products, exercise caution because the purity and processing of the substance is highly questionable and one cannot trust the methods without really knowing the entire scenario. When using natural Aloe right off the plant, make sure your use it properly, store it well and are aware of all the factors of good use.

- If you are diabetic, do not start Aloe medication oral or otherwise without your doctor's consent because it has known hypoglycemic qualities and one can lose sugar balance if sudden inflow of Aloe components happens in the blood. Also, it is not a great idea to mix medications without your doctor knowing about it.

- People with bleeding disorders, heart patients and general sensitivity, exercise caution while use and if you have a known allergy to plants of the lily family – onions and garlic and the like, better avoid Aloe too.

- Never administer even a small quantity to an infant or a child.

- When used as laxative, this might cause dependency.

Chapter 5:
A note on cultivating the Aloe plant

Well, Ayurveda bases its medications on the freshest of the fresh herbs and what can be fresher than something right off your own garden?

No, it is not as difficult as you think it is to grow Aloe Vera. This plant has certain key characteristics and if you focus on those few things, you can cultivate the Aloe Vera plant right in your backyard!

- This plant loves its sun. Plant the sapling in a sunny spot and let it grow really warm in the area. This plant thrives well in hot and arid conditions. It is quite hardy but very sensitive to cold climate.

- Water the plant with caution, as even a little extra water might kill the plant by rotting its root. Water only a little bit only when you can see cracks forming in the soil. Watch the signs of over-watering; the leaves will begin turning yellow if the plant is getting too much water. It grows exceptionally well in black cotton soil with good drainage. If possible, light soils would be good for growing Aloe Vera. It would be great if the ph balance of the soil is maintained at 8.5.

- This plant does not need any fertilizer. The roots are delicate and sensitive to change in the salt balance of the soil so avoid adding any extra fertilizers to the soil.

- When harvesting the gel, pick the last, the oldest leaf in the whorl and make a clean cut as close to the spine as possible. The thickest leaf will give more gel, as well as you will get your gel without any harm to the growing tip.

- For extracting the gel, keep the leaves facing down from the cut end to drain out all the sap or the kumarisara. This is important if you want to ingest the gel. When the sap is all drained, peel the green layer and scoop out the gel with a spoon.
- Never keep the fresh gel exposed to air or in the refrigerator for too long. Eat it as fresh as possible. For cosmetic purposes or topical application, store it in the fridge in a clean, sterile container.
- If the gel is added with vitamin E, it may stay for longer.

Cultivate the plant at home in your kitchen garden and reap the benefit of Aloe Vera fresh and nice! Only then will the effect on you be quick and efficient.

Conclusion:

"She was awake in her senses but yet to open her eyes. Her burns would sting and she would yell in pain, she thought, as the footsteps of her nurse felt closer. Swish and the sheet came off, and she prepared herself for the renewal of her wounds – she had caught fire in the kitchen in an accident and it just went out of proportion in no time. By the time she got to medical care, much had been burnt.

It was a long, painful and slow recovery. Every single day was a new torture – not once or twice but three times her wounds were exposed to the air and various concoctions applied. She would scream with the pain and had to be medicated to sleep during the early days.

She waited for the nurse to uncover her burns and put that fiery lotion on her.

Holding her breath, she waited for the substance to touch her. And it did. But surprise! It felt oddly cool and soothing… almost like watery, icy jelly – it was actually quite a nice change from that goddamn lotion.

Quietly she opened her eye. Yes, it was Aloe Vera. She would be fine soon."

Ayurveda is an ancient medical science which derives roots from the Vedas and one can find the initial records talking about how the knowledge transpired from the gods to the sages. The essence of Ayurveda is in the balance of the three doshas and their imbalance is said to cause disease. It suggests a balanced lifestyle and considers suppressing of natural desires is the cause of disease. All five senses are put to use for diagnosing a patient and the very root of the disease is found and cured. Ayurveda focuses on the prevention of a disease rather than curing it. It is a widely accepted branch of healing and more than half Indians use Ayurveda or related derived products in some form or the other in their daily life.

Ayurveda takes us through many herbs and plant products for treatment of diseases and few of them are as potent and multifunctional as the Aloe Vera plant. This plant is not just extremely versatile in applications; it is also quite common and easily accessible to most of us. This single plant has the capacity to control nearly all the systems of the body, be it immune, digestive, sensory or dermal. Owing to its many uses, most Indian homes have the Aloe plant in separate pots, placed in the sunniest part of the garden. Many kitchen gardens also house this plant for its medicinal uses.

Aloe gel is so useful, it can be applied or eaten – and it will only help your cause. From maintaining blood sugar level to regulating cholesterol, from making skin and hair healthy to curing burns, Aloe gel and juice are great plant products which are not only medicinally relevant but also nearly free!

Adding Aloe Vera to daily routine will bring about many health benefits. This coupled with proper diet will go a long way in restoring optimum health and happiness to your mind, soul and body. if the proper hygiene factors of usage are kept in mind, using Aloe Vera on a daily basis is safe and beneficial.

We hope this e-book has helped you learn more about the ayurvedic applications of Aloe Vera.

Thank you for reading!